Try It Now! GREEN SMOOTHIES "2"
by Howard Mills

Table of Contents

8. Peach Pie Avocado Green Smoothie

9. Honey Cantaloupe Green Smoothie

10. Banana Green Pea Smoothie

11. Banana Milk Chocolate Green Smoothie

12. Apple Pie Green Smoothie

13. Cilantro Cucumber Green Smoothie Recipe

14. Almond Butter Green Smoothie

15. Sweet and Sour Green Fruit smoothie

16. Sour Kiwi Lemon Green Smoothie

1. Introduction

Hello and welcome to the healthy eating lifestyle. Thank you for downloading my book. This amazing book contains a compiled list of 19 more High Quality Green Smoothie recipes that will make your taste buds dance. These Green Smoothie recipes will hold your hand and guide you down the path of healthy living. Hope you All enjoy!

2. Pink Grapefruit Green Smoothie

Pink Grapefruit and Pineapple Green Smoothie

Servings 7-8

Ingredients:

- 4 cups fresh pineapple chunks, 1¼ pounds
- 3 large pink grapefruits, 2½ pounds
- ½ ripe avocado, peeled and pitted
- 4 cups washed baby spinach, 4 ounces

Directions:

1. Place the pineapple chunks into a high powered blender.

2. Cut the grapefruits in half and juice them, discarding any large seeds.

3. Pour the grapefruit juice over the pineapple, then add the avocado and spinach.

4. Blend until completely smooth.

5. Serve immediately.

3. Banana Pina Colada Green Smoothie

Banana Pina Colada Green Smoothie

Servings 2

Ingredients:

- 1 cup coconut milk

- 2 tbsp shredded coconut (optional)

- 1 cup spinach, packed

- ½ frozen banana

- 1 cup frozen pineapple chunks

Directions:

1. Place the ingredients in a blender or food processor in the order they are listed above. Layering from liquid to frozen makes for easier blending.

2. Serve right away.

4. Avocado Re Hydration Green Smoothie

Avocado Re Hydration Green Smoothie

Servings 1-2

Ingredients:

- 1 celery stalk

- 1 small frozen banana

- half of a small avocado

- 1 gigantic handful baby spinach or other leafy green

- 1 Tbsp. plant-based protein powder

- 1/2 tsp. fresh grated ginger

- 1 cup coconut water

- juice of half a lime

Directions:

1. In a high-powered blender, blend all ingredients until completely smooth. Chill if desired. Serve.

5. Kiwi Banana Green Smoothie

Kiwi Banana Green Smoothie

Serving 1-2

Ingredients:

- 3 kiwis
- 2 bananas
- 2 nectarines
- 3 cups spinach
- 1 cup water

Directions:

1. Place all ingredients in a blender. Blend until smooth. Serve.

6. Chocolate Iron-Rich Green Smoothie

Chocolate Iron-Rich Green Smoothie

Servings 1

Ingredients:

- 1 and 1/2 oranges, peeled
- 1 banana, peeled
- 1 tablespoon cacao powder
- 2 tablespoons raw cashew nuts
- 2 cups baby spinach
- 2 ounces of water if needed (or coconut water)

Directions:

1. Start by adding the liquid to your blender, followed by the soft fruit. Add the greens to your blender last. Blend on high for 30 seconds or until the smoothie is creamy. Serve.

7. Greek Yogurt Green Spinach Smoothie

Greek Yogurt Green Spinach Smoothie

Servings 2

Ingredients:

- 1 cup Greek yogurt
- 1/2 cup water
- 1/2 cucumber
- 1 pear
- 1-2 kiwi
- 1 cup baby spinach
- 1 cup baby bok choy
- 1 cup baby kale
- 1/2-1 Tbsp raw honey

Directions:

1. Peal cucumber, pear and kiwi. Remove pear's core and remove the white part in the center of the kiwi.

2. Add Greek yogurt, water, fruit and vegetables to blender and blend on high for at least 3 minutes until all ingredients are well incorporated and smooth. Serve.

8. Peach Pie Avocado Green Smoothie

Peach Pie Avocado Green Smoothie

Servings 1-2

Ingredients:

- 1 ripe avocado

- 1 ripe peach, pitted

- 1 cup unflavored, unsweetened almond or soy milk

- 1 tbsp. agave (or to taste)

- 1 tsp. cinnamon

Directions:

1. Place all ingredients in blender and blend until smooth. Serve.

9. Honey Cantaloupe Green Smoothie

Honey Cantaloupe Green Smoothie

Servings 2

Ingredients:

- 1 cucumber, peeled and seeded

- 2 cups cantaloupe chunks (from about 1/4 large cantaloupe)

- 1 cup finely chopped kale or baby spinach leaves

- 1/4 cup fresh basil leaves

- 1/4 cup fresh mint leaves

- 3/4 cup plain unsweetened almond milk

- 1 teaspoon honey

- 1/2 teaspoon pure almond extract

Directions:

1. Combine all ingredients in a blender; blend until smooth. Pour into 2 glasses and serve.

10. Banana Green Pea Smoothie

Banana Green Pea Smoothie

Servings 1

Ingredients:

- ⅔ cup frozen peas

- 2 cups spinach

- 1 banana, preferably frozen

- ¾ cup organic apple juice

- ¼ cup coconut water (or plain water)

- 1 tablespoon chia seed or milled flax seed

- additional sweetener, as needed

Directions:

1. Place all ingredients together in the bowl of a blend and blend on high until completely smooth. Serve.

11. Banana Milk Chocolate Green Smoothie

Banana Milk Chocolate Green Smoothie

Servings 1

Ingredients:

- ¼ Cup milk

- ¾ Cup plain or vanilla yogurt

- 1 Banana

- 3 Dove Chocolates (dark) or roughly 2-3 Tbsp Chips

- 1 Cup ice

Directions:

1. Pour the milk onto the blades of the blender. Add the banana, chocolate, and yogurt and mix well. Next add ice and blend until there are no ice or chocolate pieces left then serve.

12. Apple Pie Green Smoothie

Apple Pie Green Smoothie

Servings 1

Ingredients:

- 2 Granny Smith apples, cored and sliced (not peeled)

- 1/2 cup 0% fat Greek yogurt, plain

- 1/2 cup baby spinach

- 1/4 cup quick cooking oats

- 1 tablespoon honey

- ½ teaspoon ground cinnamon

- ¼ teaspoon ground nutmeg

- 1/2 cup crushed ice

Directions:

1. Place all the ingredients into a blender and process until smooth and creamy. Taste and adjust the sweetness if necessary.

2. To serve, pour into a glass.

13. Cilantro Cucumber Green Smoothie Recipe

Cilantro Cucumber Green Smoothie Recipe

Servings 2

Ingredients:

- 1/2 cup cilantro
- 1 cup chopped cucumber
- Juice of one lime
- 2 teaspoons grated ginger
- 4 dried figs
- 4 ounces sheep or coconut yogurt

Directions:

1. Add all ingredients to a high speed blender.

2. Puree on high until completely smooth.

3. Serve immediately.

14. Almond Butter Green Smoothie

Almond Butter Green Smoothie

Servings 1

Ingredients:

- 1 tablespoons unsalted creamy almond butter

- 2 cups fresh spinach (tightly packed)

- 1 cup vanilla almond milk

- 1/2 ripe banana

- 1/4 cup frozen pineapple chunks

- Optional: 1 teaspoon chia seeds or 1 teaspoon flax seeds

Directions:

1. Combine all ingredients in a blender and blend on medium high speed until fully combined. The smoothie should be bright green and the spinach should be completely blended into the mixture then serve.

15. Sweet and Sour Green Fruit smoothie

Sweet and Sour Green Fruit smoothie

Servings 3

Ingredients:

- 1 cup coconut water or regular water (use less for a thicker smoothie)

- 1 cup of pineapple cubes

- 1 cup of green grapes

- 1 granny smith apple, cut into chunks

- 1 loosely packed cup of kale that's been torn into small pieces

- 1 cup ice

Directions:

1. Put all ingredients into your blender and blend until smooth then serve.

16. Sour Kiwi Lemon Green Smoothie

Sour Kiwi Lemon Green Smoothie

Servings 2-3

Ingredients:

- 1 large granny smith apple or any other apple of your choice

- 2 cups of spinach

- 2 kiwis peeled

- 1 lemon peeled and seeded

- 2 cups of water

Directions:

1. Peel the lemon and remove the seeds.

2. Peel the kiwis and remove seeds from apple.

3. Put lemon, kiwis, apple and spinach in a blender and process until smooth then serve.

17. Greek Sour Apple Green Smoothie

Greek Sour Apple Green Smoothie

Servings 4

Ingredients:

- 1 banana
- 1 cup Greek yogurt
- 1 tablespoon flax seeds
- 1 apple
- 1 cup orange juice
- 1/2 cup skim milk

Directions:

1. In a blender, add apple, banana, and juice. Blend until smooth. Add yogurt, milk and flaxseed oil. Blend again. Divide evenly between 4 glasses and serve.

18. Peanut Butter Banana Green Smoothie

Peanut Butter Banana Green Smoothie

Servings 1-2

Ingredients:

- 1 cup unsweetened almond or soy milk

- 1-2 handfuls of spinach

- 2 frozen bananas

- 2-4 soft pitted dates

- 2 tbsp hemp hearts

- 1 tbsp natural peanut butter

- 2 ice cubes

Directions:

1. Combine all ingredients, blend on high until perfectly smooth then serve.

19. Vanilla Lime Yogurt Green Smoothie

Vanilla Lime Yogurt Green Smoothie

Servings 1

Ingredients:

- 1/2 cup vanilla yogurt

- 1 cup spinach leaves, packed

- 2 teaspoons honey

- 1/2 banana, best frozen

- 2 tablespoons fresh lime juice

- 1/2 teaspoon pure vanilla extract

- 1/2 cup milk

- 1/2 – 1 cup ice (optional)

Directions:

1. Place all ingredients except the ice in a blender and puree until blended. Add ice and puree until smooth. Pour into a glass and serve with a straw.

20. Strawberry Green Spinach Smoothie

Strawberry Green Spinach Smoothie

Servings 2

Ingredients:

- 2 cups strawberries

- 1 banana

- 1 young coconut, water and meat

- 2 cups spinach

- 2 celery stalks

- 1-inch cube ginger, grated

- Juice of 1 lime

- 1 cup water

Directions:

1. Blend everything in blender until smooth then serve.

21. Greek Yougurt Vanilla Protien Green Smoothie

Greek Yogurt Vanilla Protein Green Smoothie

Servings 1

Ingredients:

- 1 tablespoon almond butter
- 2/3 cup Greek yogurt
- 1/2 banana
- 3/4 cup water
- 1 scoop vanilla protein powder
- 2 cups spinach

Directions:

1. Add all ingredients to blender and blend until smooth then serve.

22. Conclusion

Thank you again for downloading my recipe book. Hope you enjoy the recipes!